## DISCLAIMER

This journal is for educational and personal reflection purposes only. It is not a substitute for professional mental health care, therapy, diagnosis, or treatment. Engaging with this journal does not constitute a therapeutic relationship with Jamie Codispoti, LCSW, or Sloane Therapy Group, LLC.

If you are experiencing distress, a mental health crisis, or feel unsafe, please contact a licensed mental health professional, call 911, or reach out to the National Suicide & Crisis Lifeline at 988.

All content within this journal is protected by copyright law and is intended for personal use only. No portion of this journal may be copied, reproduced, distributed, or resold without explicit written permission from the publisher.

By using this journal, you agree to these terms and acknowledge that the content is not a replacement for professional mental health services.

If you or someone you know is in crisis, call 911 or 988 for help. This journal is not a substitute for therapy or crisis support.

For personal use only. Not for resale, commercial distribution, or duplication.
© 2025 Sloane Therapy Group, LLC.
All rights reserved.

*Hey You,*

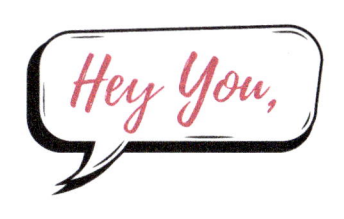

If you're holding this journal, you already know.
You've been biting your tongue. Carrying too much. Shrinking, apologizing, bending, and putting everyone else first. You've convinced yourself it's fine — that you're fine — even when your body, your energy, your gut has been telling you otherwise.

Here's the truth: pretending you're okay is exhausting. And you don't have to do it anymore.

I'm not just writing this as a therapist with 20+ years in the field. I'm writing this as someone who's sat with women unraveling in silence — and someone who's unraveled, too. I've watched women come into my office smiling on the outside, disconnected on the inside. I've seen the damage that comes from stuffing it down, making it look easy, and apologizing for needing more.

This journal is your space to say the sh*t
you've been holding in.

The thoughts you're scared to name. The feelings you've been taught are "too much." The truth you're finally ready to stand in. You don't need permission to take up space here. You don't need to earn rest or peace or clarity.
You just have to show up — as you are.
Unfiltered. Unapologetic. Unfolding.

You're not broken. You're not weak.
You're not asking for too much.

You're just finally listening to yourself.
Keep writing. Keep choosing you.

♡ Jamie
Founder of STG Wellness
Therapist. Writer. Truth teller. Firestarter.

# About STG Wellness

Hi, I'm Jamie — licensed clinical social worker, journal creator, and the unapologetic voice behind STG Wellness.

I've spent the last 25+ years helping women navigate the hardest seasons of their lives — but I've also lived them.

I've walked through divorce. I've endured devastating loss. I've experienced complicated family dynamics, fractured relationships, and the gut-punch clarity of realizing who's really in your corner when shit hits the fan.

I earned both my bachelor's and master's degrees from Florida State University. My clinical path led me from working at a high-end private school in Boca Raton to the front lines of an inpatient psychiatric hospital in Nashville. For the past two decades, I've been in private practice — sitting across from women navigating depression, anxiety, trauma, addiction, burnout, motherhood, heartbreak, and everything in between.

STG Wellness was born out of everything I've lived and everything I've witnessed in the women I've worked with.

I've sat with women who take care of everyone else before checking in with themselves. Who hold families together, lead in their careers, show up for everyone — and still feel like they've lost themselves in the process.

I've been that woman, too.

And I've also had the honor of sitting with those same women as they rebuild. I've watched the shift — when they stop apologizing for their needs, when they start using their voice, when they finally remember who they are. I've seen the power that comes from choosing yourself, and I built STG Wellness to help more women do exactly that.

We forget ourselves — not because we're weak, but because we've been conditioned to prioritize everything and everyone else.

I created STG Wellness because I wanted to build something that cuts through the noise — something bold, honest, and healing. A space where women can come back to their truth. A journal they can fill with the stuff they're afraid to say out loud. A reminder that they deserve to feel whole — not when everything else is handled, but right now. I believe in people when they don't believe in themselves. I believe in resilience, support, and taking care of yourself like your life depends on it — because sometimes it does.

And I believe in walking through life with confidence, fire, and truth — no matter what anyone else thinks about it. When someone picks up one of these journals, I hope they feel awakened. I hope they feel empowered. I hope they feel confident in their voice, bold in their healing, and grounded in who they are — not who the world told them to be.

I am so happy you are here.

Let's get started.

Jamie
**Truth-teller. Firestarter. Soul awakener.**

# No more playing small. You're allowed to take up space.

# What to Expect

Welcome to a space where you don't have to shrink, apologize, or sugarcoat your truth. This journal is here for the real you — the unfiltered, raw, healing version of you who deserves to be heard.

## Inside, you'll find:

- Daily prompts that invite you to speak the truth you've been silencing.

- Reflection questions that challenge old patterns and build new strength.

- Mindfulness tools for when the noise inside your head gets loud.

- Empowering reminders that choosing yourself is not selfish — it's necessary.

Some days you'll feel **powerful**. Some days you'll feel **cracked open.**
Both are healing.
Both are welcome.

This isn't about **perfection**. It's about **showing up** — boldly, imperfectly, and without **apology.**

# How to Use This Journal

You don't need to have it all figured out to start. This journal is your space — to feel, to process, to remember who the hell you are. Some days you'll write a lot. Some days you'll stare at the page.
Both are valid.

## Here's what to keep in mind as you move through these pages:

There's no "right" way to journal. Show up messy, honest, quiet, or bold. You don't have to make it pretty — you just have to make it yours.

Give yourself permission. Permission to rest. To rage. To dream. To not know. This space is for you, and you alone.

If something stings — pause. Growth can feel uncomfortable. Take a breath. Walk away. Come back when you're ready. Be unfiltered. These pages don't need approval. Say what you've been holding in. You're safe here.

This journal isn't about becoming someone new. It's about coming back to yourself—boldly, unapologetically, and without a damn filter.

Lean into the Reflection Pages. These aren't filler. They're your pause — your breath — your reset. Healing brings things to the surface: rage, grief, clarity, questions you didn't expect. This space was built to hold all of it. Use it to sit with what's real, to catch your breath, to stay with yourself when things get loud. You don't need a perfect answer — just the courage to keep showing up.

# Mindfulness + Breathing Techniques

When the world gets loud — when your mind races, your heart pounds, and everything feels like too much — your breath is your anchor.

## Here are simple ways to reconnect to yourself when you feel overwhelmed:

You deserve to feel steady inside your own skin.

Come back to your breath as many times as you need to.

No shame.
No apology.

## Box Breathing

- Inhale slowly for 4 counts.
- Hold your breath for 4 counts.
- Exhale slowly for 4 counts.
- Hold your breath out for 4 counts.
  (Repeat 4 times.)

## 5-4-3-2-1 Grounding

- Name 5 things you can see.
- Name 4 things you can feel.
- Name 3 things you can hear.
- Name 2 things you can smell.
- Name 1 thing you can taste.

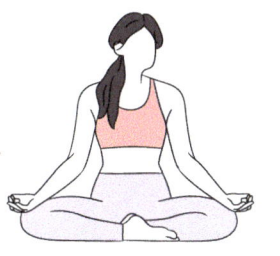

## One-Minute Reset

- Place your hand over your heart.
- Breathe in slowly, counting to 5.
- Exhale slowly, counting to 7.
- Whisper to yourself: "I am safe. I am here. I am enough."

# "Self-Compassion" Reminder

Healing isn't about being perfect. Healing isn't about getting it right every day. Healing is messy. Healing is loud sometimes. Healing is quiet sometimes. When the old patterns whisper that you're not enough, not lovable, not worthy — Answer back.
**Speak to yourself the way you would speak to someone you love.**

## Try this when the world feels heavy:

- "I'm allowed to be a work in progress."
- "My mistakes don't define me."
- "I am learning, growing, rebuilding — and that is enough."

*Choosing yourself is not selfish. It's survival. It's sacred. It's necessary. You are doing better than you know. Keep going.*

# Self-Care While Rediscovering Yourself

Because coming home to yourself can feel like losing your grip first.

Realignment isn't all candlelight and yoga. Sometimes it's crying in your car. Sometimes it's rage. Sometimes it's silence so loud it forces you to finally listen.

Rediscovering who you are — underneath the expectations, the roles, the noise — is beautiful as hell. But let's be real: it's also brutal. So here's your permission to take care of yourself like you're doing sacred, holy work. Because you are.

**This part is messy. But it's yours. Protect it. Honor it. Let it be loud. Because on the other side of this? You. Realigned. Reclaimed. Unapologetically AF.**

# Here's what real self-care can look like right now:

- Say no to anything that feels fake.
  You don't need to justify your "no." Your nervous system already gave you the answer.

- Write it out, scream it out, sweat it out.
  Movement and expression aren't optional — they're medicine.

- Give your phone a damn time-out.
  Silence the noise. Not everyone needs access to your becoming.

- Eat food that makes you feel nourished, not punished. Rediscovery requires fuel. Not restriction. Not guilt.

- Take the nap. Cancel the plan. Be unavailable.
  Rest is not laziness — it's resistance against burnout culture.

- Be around people who see you, not manage you.
  If you have to shrink to be loved, it's not love.

# Use These Tools Whenever You Need

Healing isn't linear. Some days, the prompts will crack you wide open. Some days, they'll light a fire inside you. Whenever you feel overwhelmed, anxious, or exhausted while working through this journal —

**Pause.**

Come back to your breath.
Practice the grounding techniques.
Speak to yourself with fierce self-compassion. You are allowed to take as many breaks as you need. You are allowed to feel everything without apology.

**This journal — and your healing — are both here for the messy, beautiful, real version of you.**

Where choosing yourself isn't selfish — it's powerful.

# What part of *me* am I still *silencing?*

*Let it all out. There's no right way to feel — only the truth you're finally ready to name.*

_____
_____
_____
_____
_____
_____
_____
_____
_____
_____

# Where in my *life* have I been playing *small*?

*You don't need to shrink to be accepted. Let this be the page where you expand.*

_____
_____
_____
_____
_____
_____
_____
_____
_____

# What am I really *angry* about — *underneath* it all?

*It's okay to name the hard things. You can hold space for truth and healing at the same time.*

_____
_____
_____
_____
_____
_____
_____
_____
_____

# Reflections:

- Where in my life am I ready to stop shrinking myself to make others comfortable?

- What have I been apologizing for that I actually don't owe anyone?

- When was the last time I chose peace over people-pleasing?

# Who or what have I been saying *yes* to out of *guilt*?

*This is your space to say 'no' — without apology, without explanation.*

---
---
---
---
---
---
---
---
---
---
---

# When *did* I stop trusting *myself*?

*You don't need to justify your intuition. Start listening again, one word at a time.*

_____
_____
_____
_____
_____
_____
_____
_____
_____
_____
_____
_____

# What would I *say* if I wasn't *afraid* of being *judged*?

*Let your pen say what your mouth has been holding back. You deserve to be heard.*

_____
_____
_____
_____
_____
_____
_____
_____
_____
_____

# Where have I *abandoned* my own needs?

*There's nothing selfish about wanting to feel okay again.*

_____
_____
_____
_____
_____
_____
_____
_____
_____
_____
_____

# What do I want to *reclaim* that I've *given* away?

*You get to take up space — your dreams, your time, your energy — all of it is valid.*

_____
_____
_____
_____
_____
_____
_____
_____
_____
_____

**Because choosing yourself changes everything.**

# What story about *myself* am I ready to let go of?

*Rewrite the narrative. You are not who hurt you, and you are not your past.*

# What would it look like to choose *myself* — unapologetically?

*This is your space to explore who you are when no one is telling you to dim your light.*

_____
_____
_____
_____
_____
_____

# What's *something* I've been pretending doesn't bother *me*?

*You don't have to minimize your pain to make others comfortable.*

# Where in my *life* do I feel like I'm just going through the *motions*?

*This is your invitation to wake up your truth — even if it whispers at first.*

_____
_____
_____
_____
_____
_____
_____

# What *boundary* do I wish I had the *courage* to set?

*Boundaries aren't selfish — they're sacred. Start by writing it down.*

_____
_____
_____
_____
_____
_____
_____
_____
_____
_____
_____

# Reflections:

- Where do I feel called to be bolder, louder, or more unapologetically me?

- If I could write a permission slip to myself today, what would it say?

- What does "choosing myself" look like right now, in this season of my life?

_____
_____
_____
_____
_____
_____
_____
_____
_____
_____
_____

# What's one *thing* I've been craving but afraid to ask for?

*Your needs are not too much. They are the key to your wholeness.*

___
___
___
___
___
___
___
___
___
___

# Where have I been dimming my *light* for others?

*You were never meant to shrink in order to be loved.*

_____
_____
_____
_____
_____
_____
_____
_____
_____
_____

# Who *am* I when I stop *performing*?

*Let this page be a mirror — for the real, raw, powerful version of you.*

_____
_____
_____
_____
_____
_____
_____
_____
_____
_____
_____
_____
_____

# What part of *me* am I proud of, even if no one *sees* it?

*You don't need applause to be worthy. You get to be proud — out loud.*

_____
_____
_____
_____
_____
_____
_____
_____
_____
_____
_____

# When did I *first* learn that my voice didn't matter?

*That was a lie. Your words hold weight. Let them out here.*

_____
_____
_____
_____
_____
_____
_____
_____
_____
_____
_____

# Say what you're afraid to say out loud.

# What's *something* I've forgiven others for, but haven't forgiven *myself* for?

*You deserve the same grace you give to everyone else.*

# What truth do I *keep* shoving down to keep the *peace*?

*Keeping the peace shouldn't cost you your own.*

# Where in my *life* am I still waiting for *permission*?

*Permission doesn't come from others. It starts with you.*

_____
_____
_____
_____
_____
_____
_____
_____
_____
_____
_____
_____

# What am I tired of *explaining* to people who don't get it?

*You don't have to justify your truth. Not everyone deserves access to it.*

# What do I *wish* someone would *finally* acknowledge?

*Even if no one else says it — write it for yourself. You've carried so much.*

_____
_____
_____
_____
_____
_____
_____

# Reflections:

- What boundaries do I need to set to protect my peace, energy, and identity?

- What parts of me feel the most powerful, and how can I honor them more?

- Who do I become when I stop seeking permission to be who I am?

# Where have I been *over-functioning* to feel worthy?

*Your value is not based on how much you produce or fix for others.*

# What *truth* about *myself* scares me — and excites me?

*That feeling? That's growth.
Let yourself explore it safely here.*

# What am I ready to let go of — even if it still *hurts*?

*Healing doesn't require perfection.
It begins with release.*

_____
_____
_____
_____
_____
_____
_____
_____
_____
_____

# What would I say if I *believed* I was already enough?

*This page knows your worth — now write like you do too.*

_____
_____
_____
_____
_____
_____
_____
_____

# How have I *made* myself smaller to make *others* feel bigger?

*You don't have to shrink to coexist.*
*You were meant to take up space.*

_____
_____
_____
_____
_____
_____
_____

# Reflections:

- Where am I tired of explaining myself, and what will I do about it?

- What parts of myself have I hidden to be accepted — and why?

- What would it look like if I lived completely unapologetically for one day?

**You don't need permission. You need a pen.**

# What would I do *differently* if I wasn't afraid of *being misunderstood*?

*Misunderstood doesn't mean wrong. It means brave.*

_____
_____
_____
_____
_____
_____
_____
_____

# What's something I need to say — and to whom — even if they *never* read it?

*Say it here. Say it loud. This space was made for your voice.*

_____
_____
_____
_____
_____
_____
_____
_____

# This is not the watered-down version of you.

# Reflections:

- Where am I still waiting for validation that I don't actually need?

- How would my life change if I trusted myself as much as I trust others?

- What am I most proud of — even if no one else sees it?

Your truth is not too much. It's just not for everyone.

# 30 / 60 / 90-Day Goals: The No Apologies Way

This isn't about fixing yourself.
It's about finally showing up for yourself —
with honesty, fire, and zero apologies.

Let this be the moment you stop shrinking
and start choosing you

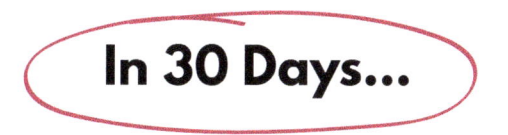

## In 30 Days...

**I will stop apologizing for:**

_____
_____
_____
_____
_____

**I will start honoring this truth about myself:**

_____
_____
_____
_____

**I will give less energy to:**

_____
_____
_____
_____

**I will make space for:**

_____
_____
_____
_____

**Keep going — this is your firestarter.**

## In 60 Days...

### I will speak up when:

___

### I will say "no" to:

___

**I will say "hell yes" to:**

_____
_____
_____
_____
_____
_____
_____

**I will feel most proud of:**

_____
_____
_____
_____
_____
_____
_____

# Look at you — unlearning the bullshit and owning your life.

# In 90 Days...

**I will be unapologetic about:**

_____
_____
_____
_____
_____
_____

**I will rewrite this belief that's been holding me back:**

_____
_____
_____
_____
_____
_____

**I will show up for myself by:**

_____
_____
_____
_____
_____
_____

**This is the version of me I'm stepping into:**

_____
_____
_____
_____
_____

# You're not becoming someone else. You're coming back to you.

## Before You Go...

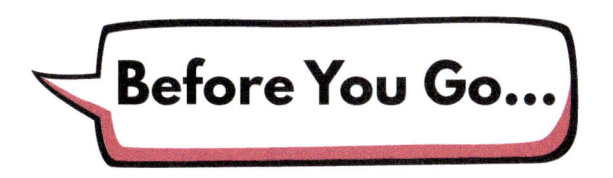

### You made it.

Thirty days of truth-telling, boundary-setting, and choosing yourself.

That's not small. That's not soft. That's power.

You didn't just fill up a journal — you showed up for yourself. You told the truth. You didn't water it down. And that matters more than you know.

If your pages look a little messy — good. If your words were hard to write — even better. That means you're doing the work most people avoid their whole damn lives.

**This isn't the end. It's the beginning.
Of you** — **unfiltered. Unapologetic. On fire.**

## So what's next?

You keep going.
You speak louder.
You stop shrinking.

You take up space — and then some.

And when the world tells you to quiet down?

You write louder.
You heal louder.
You live louder.

Because choosing yourself isn't selfish —
it's necessary.

And you, my friend, are just getting started.

## With all the fire,
♡ **STG** Wellness

**P.S.**

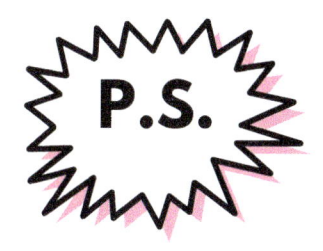

If this journal cracked something open, you're not alone. Check out our other STG Wellness journals — created to help you dig deeper, reconnect with yourself, and keep choosing your truth:

## STG Wellness Journals :

✓ **Back To Me: 30 Days to Remember Who the Hell I Am.**

✓ **Aligned As Hell: Where Your Fire Meets Your Truth.**

✓ **The Reintroduction: Unfiltered. Aligned. Unapologetically Me.**

Find Us On Etsy | Stgwellness.etsy.com

You don't have to do this alone.
We're building a movement —
one bold page at a time.